I was Addicted to this Drug

How 'bout You?

Robert Billions Kincade III

Demetrice Kincade Sheriff, M.A.Ed.

Disclaimer

This book was written with the sole purpose of helping people. It is not meant to dictate to people to replace anything they desire to eat. We are not doctors; however, the information we share can be very helpful for the mind, body, and soul.

Don't get us wrong. We thank God for hospitals and doctors because we do need them, but we could need them much less if we would educate ourselves.

Published by CLF Publishing, LLC. 3281 Guasti Road, Seventh Floor, Ontario, CA 91761. (760) 669-8149.

Cover Design by Senir Design. Contact information- info@senirdesign.com.

Photographers- Rod Goodman (for Robert Kincade's photo on the front cover and Demetrice Kincade Sheriff's photo on the back cover).

ISBN # 978-1-4675-6883-8

Printed in the United States of America.

Appreciations

To anyone out there who opened up this book and gave me a chance as a writer it means a lot. I would like to say you are allowing my dreams to come true. To anyone who enjoys my work, I promise to have future materials for you to read.

I appreciate my internal family for supporting anything that I do that is positive. Love all of you. This is a new beginning for all of us.

Robert

To my daughter, Cherice, and nephew, Robert IV, who I love abundantly, I appreciate you both for your continued support.

Demetrice

We appreciate our deceased grandparents, our grandmother, aunts, uncles, cousins, family and friends. We love you all and thank you for your support.

We truly appreciate our parents Robert and Bettie Kincade for being the best. We love you!!!

Robert & Demetrice

Thanks

Thank you God for making this possible.

Thank you to my manager who happens to be my sister Demetrice (AKA Mica) for all the great effort and energy behind our first project together. Looking forward to working with you on many great future projects. You know I have a lot of wild and crazy ideas. There is great fun ahead of us!

Thank you to my dad for helping me create the book cover.

Thank you to Rod Goodman for the photos.

Special thanks

My sister and I both would like to thank Dr. Cassundra White-Elliott of CLF Publishing, LLC for her hard work and dedication. She is the reason this project was able to happen so quickly. Cassundra, you are an amazing person!

Table of Contents
Volume 1

Table of Contents
Volume 2

Volume 1

Chapter 1

For the Love of the Gym

The year was 2001, when I first had thoughts about lifting weights. Growing up as a teenager, I was always the skinny handsome guy. Although this was not a bad thing, I looked like a normal but slender man when I reached adulthood. I started to debate if I wanted to continue to look the same or try something new.

At the time, I had very little money to join a gym, so I decided to settle for an old weight set I had lying around in the garage that was begging to be dusted off. It was filthily disgustingly dusty. After the big clean-up, I had about 80 pounds of weights to work with. At the time, I thought that was a large amount of iron to be lifting. Doing the bench press with 50 pounds was murder to my little chest.

Just the thought of working out made me feel good inside, and working out is not complete without some form of exercise to get the good old heart pumping. Basketball always had been a huge part of my life, and that was all the cardio conditioning I needed. The problem was I was not playing basketball often like I did in the past. Jogging was the only thing that came into my mind. Over time, I knew this combination would pump out some good results.

Two days a week, I would do my workouts. It was not bad doing a few curls for the arms. I finished off with a slow run around the block. After a short period of time, I stopped being afraid of the dreadful bench press. This activity would go on time after time over the next couple of years.

As time kept flying, the year 2005 was here. Simply staying in shape was not cutting it anymore. Once again, I was no longer satisfied with my physique. When I looked in the mirror, I was in shape, but I was still too thin above my waist. Every time I would be in a store, a bodybuilding magazine would find its way into my hands. I couldn't take it anymore. It was time to join a gym.

The only thing holding me back was that I could not afford the payments for the gym. The laws of attraction were on my side because sure enough my sister gave me a call one day asking if I was interested in getting a gym membership. I had to jump on this deal right away because she worked for a corporation that gave huge discounts for 24hour Fitness. I told her to sign me up the next day.

Joining the gym was a bit intimidating at first. My first time there I did not know what the heck to do besides giving a lucky lady a chance at having a future date with me (LOL). Plus, I didn't know how to use half the equipment. I did not want to ask anyone for assistance, especially a female because that would give the perception that I was a rookie. As we all know, men have a stupid ego problem at times. So, I basically did a lot of watching until I was not intimidated by the machines anymore.

Once I found a routine that was comfortable, it was time for me to develop some muscles. I raised the bar by going from two days a week to four days a week to the gym. The months would zoom by and the fitness world would now become part of my life. It's true what people say, "It can be addicting." Sometimes, I would get upset if I couldn't make it to the gym.

My reflection in the mirror was starting to show some results, but satisfaction was not met. I was tired of seeing the muscle-bound guys strutting around laughing all the time. I wanted to be one of them. The icing on the cake was when I would be at home watching videos and see a guy like LL Cool J shirtless living it up in the rap videos.

So how would I get bigger? I was not too thrilled about taking all the protein powders, so I decided to shoot up a few steroids that I purchased on the black market. (Just kidding.) I decided to start powering down more food. You know eating is an addiction in itself. Constantly, I would eat everything, especially if it was said to be high in protein. I was not normally a big beef eater, but during that time, I probably became half cow.

By 2007, I had packed on about 25 pounds, which made a tremendous difference. I didn't get on the scale a lot back then, but my clothes fit differently. Many people started questioning me about what I was doing or taking. Guys were asking me pointers about weight lifting, and women would just ask questions just to be asking. Ladies really do dig muscles, which will never change. During this time, I was walking into the gym with my head up high. No longer was I the rookie walking around nervously. One of the goals in my life had been accomplished. I was feeling unstoppable.

Chapter 2

Eating for Health

Like I said earlier, I was eating everything in front of me; however, that is not exactly good even though I ate plenty of vegetables and fruits. I knew this was important for health, but I didn't realize how much at the time. Although I felt good, I started to understand it was necessary for me to lower my meat intake because it was hard on the system. The result of this was a slight decrease in weight. That was not a big deal, I still maintained my guns. The one with the guns has plenty of fun.

As usual, I was still dissatisfied with my appearance. I learned part of the addiction of working out is you are never satisfied. While seeking a new look, it was time to change my eating habits, and I had to decide what not to eat because the worst food I was eating was in the form of sweets. Yes, I said sweets. This seems to be the worst nightmare of everyone. I'm not sure about the other countries, but in America, we are dessert freaks.

Since childhood, dessert has been my favorite food of the day. Like most of us, I was raised to have something sweet after every big meal. I was so brainwashed with this thought that it was hard for me to eat a meal unless I knew it would be followed by something full of sugar. Similar to most of us, I was a fanatic.

The one thing about me is I love to experiment. I was looking forward to a new challenge. I wanted to test myself mentally by trying to go without my addiction for a while. How hard could it be to put down a piece of cake for a bowl of freshly cut pineapples? How hard could it be to throw a soda in the trash can in **exchange for a cup of juice?** This sounded easy, so I decided to start drinking more water on a regular basis. After a couple of weeks of torture, I was down to drinking just one soda or soft drink per day. It was really difficult to drink water with certain foods, such as a burger and fries. Mentally, we get so conditioned into thinking that certain foods need to be combined with some kind of soft drink. This kind of thinking is pure madness. I know people think this way because many people have shared these thoughts with me. We never understand how addicted we are to something until we stop doing it. This was the beginning stage for me in figuring out how our sugar consumption is a disease.

It would be a while before my mind would allow me to drink water with any meal. It was a good feeling making it to this point. Soon, I would recognize how my body was being affected by water. No longer would I get that bloating feeling inside my stomach that I was used to. **My body felt more at peace with itself.** What I really liked was that my food would digest easier. As you all know, easy digestion means one has a much more peaceful time in the restroom. Please everyone, do yourselves a favor and more drink water.

At the gym, I would weigh myself about once a week. To my surprise, my weight went down once again. It was shocking, but I had dropped about 5 more pounds. Just from drinking water, I had lost 7 pounds total. My body mass went down a little, but it wasn't too noticeable. I continued with my same food regime, except I wanted to try resisting sweets altogether for a while. This sort of challenge would turn into a war inside my head.

I can clearly remember going two days without sugar, and I could not resist anymore. At night, I literally ran to the kitchen as if I was looking for a drug fix. To my sadness, no sweet treats were found. One might say I was really pissed off. I do not even like candy, but I shoved a couple of jelly beans in my mouth that were lying at the bottom of a jar. I spit them out because I hate jellybeans. Next, I grabbed a soda out the refrigerator and drank half of it. It did not satisfy me, but at least it calmed my sugar rush, so I could go to bed.

The next day, I bought a donut just so my mind could rest. The first few bites of that glaze donut tasted like something from heaven. After this slip up, I was ready to get back to my goal. I was beginning to think to myself the goal I had in mind would not be worth it. Dealing with sugar cravings would be too much of a monster to conquer.

The food I gave up eating was almost half my regular food intake. Giving up cereal in the morning was a very difficult food to give up. I'm sure some of you are thinking why I stopped eating cereal. Most cereal comes packed with sugar, and of course, if the cereal does not come packed with sugar, most of us dump clumps of sugar into our bowls. What was even harder than giving up cereal was giving up dessert after dinner. Sometimes, I would have to keep myself busy just to stop thinking about the sugar rage inside me. The strange thing was I started to eat less since I tried to stay away from anything with a significant amount of sugar in it.

What I found very surprising during this stage were my **emotional swings**. I was actually easy to become irritated. And anyone who knows me can tell you I am normally a calm natured person. My body and my mind were going through some serious withdrawals. A few people even asked me why I was snapping at them so much. I would jokingly play it off. Later on, I would find all the reasons behind my behavior patterns.

Chapter 3

Losing 20 Pounds in 25 Days

One day, I went to the gym and the weights felt extra heavy. I sat down for a few minutes wondering what happened to all my strength. It wasn't hard to figure out once I rushed to the scale to see how much I weighed. My weight had decreased by another 6 pounds. Wow, after a little over three weeks, I had dropped around 13 pounds. Now I wasn't expecting this, so I didn't know the kind of reactions I would get from everyone. Of course, I didn't get a great response from the heavy lifters in the gym. They thought I was committing sin by losing so much mass; however, I got a good response from pretty much everyone else. A lot of women would give me compliments for no reason. I would think to myself, *do I really look that different after all?* Many people would tell me how young I looked.

Most people really do look more youthful when they drop weight. Many women would tell me how handsome I was. The reason was simple: I had lost weight in my face. Little did I know I had found an entirely different reason to walk around with a smile on my face.

As a few more days rolled by, I noticed all my clothes were too big. My belt didn't even fit anymore. Lifting weights had now become an enemy because everything felt heavy. I hopped on the scale again to see if I had lost any more weight. To no surprise, I had dropped another 7 pounds. What would be the reaction from everyone now?

All the compliments I was getting turned against me in a flash. The ladies were asking me if I was sick. Some even offered to cook for me (LOL). At least those comments made me laugh. Many friends asked me what was I so stressed out over. For the first time, I could now look in the mirror and see how much I had changed. It was at this moment I decided to stop the madness.

I could not take it anymore. I felt good, but I was thin as a rail. Being down to 180 pounds was never a goal of mine. It was time to put back on some weight. Little did I know all this caused other problems. My stomach had shrunk to the point where I seldom had hunger pains. How was I going to put back on all that weight in a hurry? Over the next couple of weeks, I tried consuming more food. This did not work out to well because I was basically forcing myself to eat. I did not want to become a huge meat eater again, so I decided to put my body through another experiment. The next experiment would be to start putting different kinds of refined sugar into my body.

Not to my knowledge, at this point, my taste buds were highly activated. I can distinctly remember trying to eat a piece of my mom's yellow cake one evening. It was delicious, but it was too sweet. After a few mouthfuls, I was stunned because my teeth started to burn slightly. The rest of my piece of cake ended up in the trash can. By the way, my teeth burned slightly for about five minutes.

Two days later, I tried to drink a soda. I will never forget that day in my life! After drinking half the can, I started cussing out loud while I kept grabbing my cheeks! The best way I could describe this would be **like getting your teeth cleaned and you feel your gums being torn.** By the way, the burning sensation lasted about half an hour. Juices had a similar effect on me. It took a little over two weeks of constant intake of refined sugar before the sensors in my mouth stopped detecting how sweet certain foods really are.

It took about a month before I saw my weight increase from eating refined sugar along with starch-based foods. As a matter of fact, I was able to get back to about 190 pounds a few weeks later. All these weight changes happened as a result of all the processed sugars. I will never forget the lesson I learned in those three months. Refined sugar will always call my name, but I eat less sugar now than all of my years on this earth. I must say, I haven't felt this good since my high school years.

I am thankful for going through this strange process of going up and down in weight. It was because of this that I became so motivated in studying about this dreadful food we call sugar. It is truly our worst enemy. What I truly enjoy is the fact that I have not had a weight issue since.

Chapter 4

This is a Drug

I began listening to various health experts and watching food documentaries. By the time I started looking up this information in books at the library and book store, I already knew the tragedy this food was causing to us. The most stunning factor of all the information I obtained was the fact that sugar is used as a weapon against us.

This weapon happens to be the most powerful drug in the world.

Now don't get me wrong. Our bodies do need certain amounts of sugar levels to maintain good health. There is no doubt about it. The problem is people do not understand that the only sugars we need are natural sugars, which come from vegetables and fruit. Processed sugars don't grow out of the ground. It is man who creates this poison.

The harmful effects caused by sugar are countless. We get sick and end up in the hospital. The doctors tell us that we have hereditary diseases. People, we are being played like puppets. The truth is they simply cannot give a correct answer on our illness. In most cases, they don't tell us exactly how to get rid of our problems for good. By the way, the hospital is a huge monopoly game being played on all of us, but that is another topic in itself.

We need to cleanse our minds of all the brain washing we have been under for so many decades. The main doctor in your life should be you. **For it is you who controls what goes into your big mouth.** Whatever we put in our mouths determine the conditions of our bodies. From my short time of research, I have found that most people are addicted to white sugar. This sugar is a gateway to all other sugars.

Sugar is the reason most people are overweight. I had so many withdrawals because refined sugar is comparable to taking any powerful street or medical drug. You can accept this or not. Please, do your own research. My snappy attitude came about because I was not getting my usual hit of my favorite drug. We have all seen how crappy people can act when they cannot get a hold of a particular drug. The funny part is we are just as bad as they are, but we don't have a clue of what is really going on. If people were to examine themselves closely, they would see how much of a junkie they really are. Oh yes, I'm talking about all of us. The reason why we don't detect how sweet certain foods are because all the sugar we consume desensitizes all our detectors inside our bodies. **Our mouths are loaded with hundreds of sensors that are supposed to detect how harmful something is to us.**

The point I'm really trying to get across to America is that our main enemy is sugar. I tell people all the time if they are counting calories than they are possibly taking the wrong approach towards food. The calorie count is very deceptive. It is the sugar that adds up to the real calories because it does not travel through our bodies correctly. Sugar cakes up in the intestines causing constant constipation. It contaminates the blood resulting in hardening of the arteries. In the end, this potent chemical makes every organ overwork itself.

Today, I laugh when I hear someone bragging about a product that has low calorie content. But that product tastes extremely sweet. This is where I would have to say the food industry is a straight out lie in my opinion. The high sugar content mixed with chemicals is the hidden calories people need to worry about. Truthfully, the calorie count is a pure mystery. People wonder why they continue to gain weight after using these so-called fabulous products. To make matters worse is many of these chemical sugars are not even digested by our bodies. They simply pass through our intestines unprocessed. This is exactly why certain products say no calories on their labels. The food administration allows them to word it this way. If certain materials pass through our bodies unprocessed, it is labeled as empty calories. This is pure nonsense.

Sugar-free products are also brainwashing. This is a huge joke. It's merely a marketing scheme in my opinion. Usually at the core of these products is a chemically sweet taste. This goes out to you faithful sports drinkers. People fall for these gimmicks because they are packed with vitamins. I believe this gives people a false sense of energy. It's actually a sugar boost, which people keep mistaking for energy. Most of these products contain saccharin and sorbitol. I would rather have white sugar in my veins than some sort of artificial sweeteners any day. The next time you drink something sweet that has the label sugar free, I want you to ask yourself a question. How in the hell did it get sweet then?

Sugar-free products are made in laboratories. All diabetic people should be very weary of these products. A game is being played on you in my opinion. Your body is going to pay for it as well as your pockets. Diabetic cases have doubled in the last 25 years because of these kinds of artificial sweeteners.

Here is a short list of names that refined sugar is classified under. They are always lurking on the back of products in the ingredients section.

White sugar

Brown sugar

Sucrose

Beat sugar

Syrup

Molasses

Raw sugar

Invert sugar

Powdered sugar

Honey

Yes, I did say honey because it has the same effect as sugar but at a slower pace. I bet most of you say honey is great for the body. They process this delicious product also. What's funny is people think that honey just grows naturally in a comb. The truth is honey is bee saliva, or we might even want to call it bee throw up; however, it is much more nutritious if it is wild honey that is unprocessed. **But** at the end of the day, I would say raw honey has some great minerals in it, and it is used for many eating disorders.

For all you fancy drinkers out there who love sugar-free beverages containing ascorbic acid, you are being deceived in my opinion. This is worse than white sugar. The companies don't tell us this is an acid sugar.

For everyone out there who has to have a hot cup of java in the morning, which happens to be a drug in itself (but we are not discussing that), everywhere we go, we are offered sweeteners, such as Sweet 'N Low or saccharin. Pour in the white sugar over these artificial sweeteners. These kinds of chemicals produce much more damage to our bodies. You might wake up with split personalities or a nose growing on the side of your neck. Keep in mind you should be drinking coffee like the old school did with no sugar at all. **Sugar is the reason we are overweight.** Everyone should do a little research on refined sugar. You will find that it is a pretender food. They have a very low count of vitamins or minerals. The strong cells try to correct the problem in your blood stream. The end result is a depletion of our cells in general. Sugar zaps the vitamins in our bodies that should be used at a later time. This leaves the body in a state of disease. Diseases, such as sugar diabetes, heart failure, kidney failure, and all major diseases, are linked to processed sugar.

Perhaps the most notorious disease linked to sugar is the disease labeled sugar diabetes. Sugar damages the pancreas, which is the producer of insulin. When the pancreas can no longer produce insulin itself, the body gets out of order. The sugar levels in the body rocket sky high or drop far below the necessary levels. These imbalances produce symptoms such as fatigue, nervousness, irritation, and irrational thinking. These symptoms can be reversed by changing food consumption alone. If people would only take the time to study, they would find out the truth behind most of these horrible diseases. We would not have to pop pills from the doctor everyday, which do not get rid of the entire disease in the body. If they did, why would we have to continuously keep taking the pills?

Chapter 5

It's in Everything

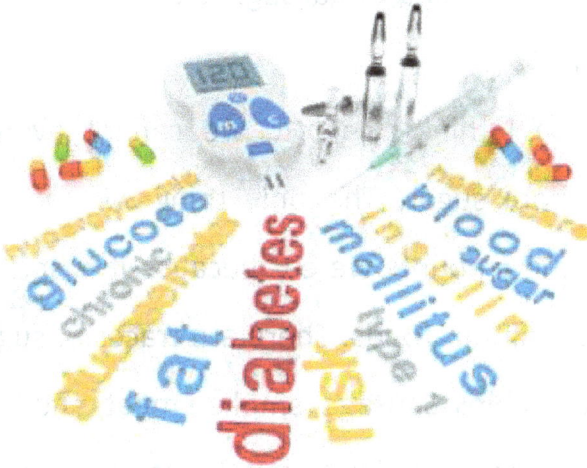

We all have times of what is called the sugar blues. It has an ancient history, but it was not a big problem until the last couple hundred years. Countless amounts of people have died involving the trade of slaves for sugar. There were plantations built to produce this evil chemical. What was once a great delicacy has become a weapon for power. It is aimed at different groups of people for mental slavery. I found it disturbing that my parents said in the past the doctors would tell them to give sugar water to their kids for energy. What kind of garbage is that? This is pure insanity.

When I think about it, we cannot even get away from sugar. The only thing we can do is lower the amounts we eat because it is sprinkled in over half our foods. There are traces of sugar in crackers, chips, sausage, smoked meat, and bread. It is not hard to figure out there is a group of people who don't care about the health issues in America. **In my opinion, it should not be in most of our foods unless we decide to put it in there.** There are far too many products in the stores loaded with sweeteners. It is bad enough that pasta and rice is nothing but starch. These are our favorites, but they do the same thing as sugar in the bloodstream.

We constantly see on television that in America there is a concern for obesity with our kids. I think back to when I was a kid in school. The snack machines would be full of candy bars and beverages. How are these products on many school campuses? Does the food administration really care about us? I would have to say no because sugar has the same effect as drugs. **It makes our bodies weak.** If your body is weak, your mind becomes weak. Drugs are used to control the thought patterns of people. There is a group of people out there who want us hooked on this stuff.

There needs to be a change in the way food is approached, but that can only be done if the kids are being taught by their parents and teachers. For decades now, we have been on a diet of foods that does not agree with our internal organs. Sugar is at the top of the pyramid when it comes to disease-causing foods.

All people have to do is write down every day for a few days what they consume. I guarantee it is mostly sugar, meat, and starch. I call these **The Big Three,** and they are all killing our systems. All people have to do is change what they eat for health. Create miracles within your own body.

I also advise people to stop eating their biggest meal at dinner time. Too many people eat too much then lay down miserably. Eat more in the day time, so your food will digest naturally from your activities throughout the day. Our eating habits are far too close to that of pigs. Instead of eating to get full, we stuff ourselves until we have no choice but to sit down for long periods of time. This is disgusting. **Let's make a change people.**

A Few Artificial Sweeteners

Saccharin

Aspartam

Sucralose

Neotame

Potassium Sorbate

Dextrose

Equal

Sorbitol

I do not tell people to stop eating refined sugar. I ask them how much sugar they put in their bodies. It is funny because every person I ask really does not know how many items are under the refined sugar umbrella. For instance, many people tell me they do not really even like sweets. I say that is good, but then I ask them what do they drink. Most of the time their favorite drink is full of high fructose corn syrup. They are shocked when I explain to them that their addiction might be worse than most people's.

All of us are in the same boat when it comes to our desire for sweets. We have not been taught the knowledge of what is in our foods. Study for yourself a little at a time, and you will see why we have so many health problems. Teach yourselves; then, teach your kids. Most of all use your common sense.

Soda- Now everyone knows this is not a product that should be consumed on a regular basis. We all know it is not good for us, but it is delicious. The problem is we drink it on a regular basis. This product has always put our bodies in a disease state, but why is it so much worse for us than it used to be?

If we look back in time before the 1980's, soda was mostly made with table sugar. Gradually, it switched from table sugar to high fructose corn syrup. This syrup is three times as sweet as table sugar. Not only that, it is much cheaper to make. The soda companies could now make twice the profit off of its consumers. Everyone was happy because there would be soda for everyone in America, and everyone could consume many varieties of soda.

A few years later, multiple health issues arose on the scene. Many people ended up in the hospitals nationwide from different diseases. They were not new, but the speed of the diseases had tripled. Perhaps the organ it did the most damage on was the liver.

My question is, "Why is soda available everywhere I look?" As an example, on many school campuses, soda and candy bars are available every day. This doesn't make sense to me. Somebody does not care about our kids. I will say though, changes are occurring on many school campuses where they are providing healthier foods.

Diet Soda- Let this be a red flag for you ladies and gentlemen. Many of you out there think this is a good replacement to drinking regular soda. The word *diet* makes the product innocent, so I understand why this sounds confusing. It is confusing. Pay close attention to the ingredients on the label. You can hardly pronounce the names of the ingredients and all chemicals. If you try to lose weight with heavy consumption of diet soda, you are in for an awakening. The ingredients are all chemicals. In fact, you are better off drinking regular sodas in my opinion.

Juices- I know many of you out there indulge in drinking juice daily because they are loaded with vitamins. It is time to break some hearts, especially you orange juice drinkers out there. Most varieties of juices are made from concentrates. But most people do not know what concentrates are. They are made from a boiling process and mostly all the healthy materials are removed. Yet, the food administration allows these products to be labeled as all natural or sugar free. It is all a game, from which these companies are getting rich. For the juices that say 25 to 50 percent real juice, you might as well drink a soda. These products contain harmful ingredients.

To people out there trying to lose weight, please do not drink large quantities of these sorts of juices. The other kind of sugar in fruit drinks is high fructose corn syrup, which is deadly. Years ago, I would drink a large cup size of different juices every morning. Over a period of time, I noticed my stomach would have a burning sensation every morning. The reason for this was everything I drank contained fructose corn syrup, which is very acidic.

To the weight watchers, keep these drinks to a minimum. The only juices that are safe in my opinion are freshly squeezed. The juices that are second in line are flash pasteurized for they contain strong traces of vitamins. The problem is this kind of juice is expensive, so don't kill yourself trying to purchase these items. No one needs a lot of juice for health anyway. Eat a piece of fruit and stop being fooled by the industry. The juices you have been drinking are just another form of sugar.

Sports Drinks/Energy Drinks- Most of them are loaded with very high sugar levels. Keep them to a minimum. The energy drinks are a new phenomenon that is putting us in the hospital at an alarming rate in my opinion. Companies keep adding chemicals we have never heard of to the products, and we cannot even pronounce them. These chemicals are tearing our bodies as well as our minds in half.

Bottom Line- Remember, we are all addicted to sugar. The lesson to be learned is lower your refined sugar intake. I still love sodas, cakes, and pies; however, I drink and eat them in moderation. My weight and my symptoms of most illnesses have stabilized. This book is dedicated to all those who are plagued by multiple health problems. Most likely your problems are coming straight from your kitchen. Wake up and smell the coffee without the sugar. You can change; I know I have.

I don't know if it's true or not until I do further studies, but some say sugar is heavily linked to fear inside the mind. This may be true because in my dreams since childhood I would always find myself being chased by someone or something. Since I stopped eating so much sugar, my dreams have changed. No longer do I run away in my dreams; now, I fight back.

What do you think?

Sugar is the worst drug in America, in my opinion. We all have friends and family that are hooked on street drugs or medical drugs. But ask yourself how many people you know are hooked on sugar. After reading the information in this book, your answer should be everyone you know, including yourself. It is true; we crave it from sunrise to sundown. By any means necessary, we make sure we get our daily boost just to get through the day.

I am not a doctor, nor do I have a medical degree, but common sense is the highest degree one can ever receive in life. I want people to know they have options. I just want to help people out a little, and that is probably why people call me a spiritual writer.

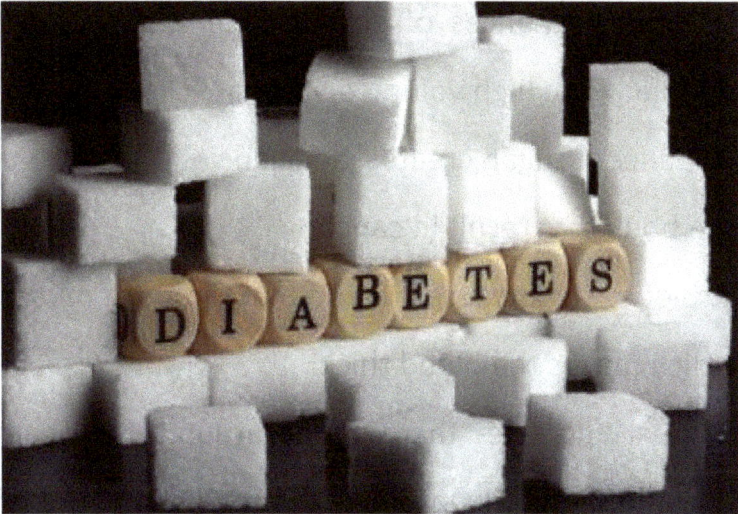

Harmful Hints of Sugar

1. Obesity- weight gain from empty calories of sugar. Sugar has almost no vitamins, minerals, or fiber.

2. Diabetes- damages the pancreas resulting in high or low sugar levels.

3. Acid reflux- sugar causes indigestion. The body in whole is put in an acid state.

4. Osteoporosis- higher sugar level can cause the bones to become soft because of low calcium levels.

5. Kidney- chances of getting kidney stones are doubled with high volumes of sugar.

6. Cancer- sugar creates deficiencies throughout the body that result in cancer.

7. Blood- sugar causes the body to produce mucus which makes the blood thick.

8. Heart disease- the arteries around the heart become clogged; therefore, the correct amount of blood doesn't flow to the heart.

9. Tooth decay- the smooth enamel on the teeth becomes scratchy. Also causes cavities and bad breath.

10. Liver- high fructose corn syrup is one of the main enemies of the liver. It causes the disease called cirrhosis, which is a contaminated liver.

Healthy Eating Tips

Start today- you're only cheating yourself by waiting until tomorrow.

Drink water- perhaps the most important part of good health. It will help wash out all the garbage you are taking in.

Sugar habits- use your common sense, please. If you have been eating cake today, don't follow it up with a soft drink. Drink water for the rest of the day. If you have been drinking soda all day, don't eat dessert.

Small portions- eat to receive energy and to be comfortable. Stop eating like it's your last meal of the day.

When to eat- there isn't a certain time to eat, but stop waiting until night to eat your biggest meal. Eat the big meal in the daytime.

Sweat- don't sit around without doing anything physical all day. Go dancing, bowling, play basketball, or join a gym. Stop making excuses.

Replace white items- replace white bread with any dark colored bread. Lower your intake of white rice and tortillas. Start eating whole grain products.

Alternatives- try maple syrup or agave syrup, raw honey, or Stevia.

Common sense- the greatest alternative

Refined Sugar Facts

1. In the early nineteenth century, it was considered to be elegant to have a bowl of sugar cubes in your kitchen.

2. The more sugar you consume, the more you crave it. One kind of sugar is a gateway to other sugars.

3. The nutritional value of sugar is almost nonexistent.

4. It is proven to make any bad health condition worse.

5. It dehydrates the body.

6. Numerous studies show that the higher amount of sugar people consume, the more weight they will gain.

7. Hidden sugars are found in chips, bread, juices, sports drinks, etc.

8. Sugar is the main reason people spend so much money whenever they enter the grocery stores.

We are unconsciously attracted to anything that looks sweet.

Definitions

Refined sugar- process of extracting the sucrose from a particular plant. The water content is removed along with other materials. The vitamins and fibers are inside these materials.

Sucrose- organic compound known as table sugar. Also called table sugar, white sugar, brown sugar, turbinated sugar, invert sugar, cane sugar, beet sugar, and saccharose.

Molasses- a by-product of sugar refining. It is produced as a sweet thick liquid.

Concentrate- Concentrated fruit juice has all the water content removed. The water is what contains all the mineral contents. What is left is a sweet substance, which is harmful when taking in large amounts.

Black strap molasses- a by-product of molasses. It is produced as a dark thick liquid.

Artificial sweeteners- a food additive that duplicates the effects of sugar in taste with a lot less energy.

High fructose corn syrup- sugar made from a highly processed corn. Should be called corn sugar.

Drug- a substance once absorbed into the body alters normal bodily functions.

Diabetes- a serious disease caused by high levels of sugar in the blood. Curable by changing diet habits.

Testimony:

Robert is my younger brother. I have so much respect for him. Over the last few years, he has earned a doctorate in life in my opinion. A few years ago, I gained weight and could not get the weight off for nothing. I would work out at the gym and lose inches, but the scale remained the same. In a conversation with my brother, I was explaining my frustrations. I explained to him what I ate and drank daily. He said to try to take sugar out of my diet. He went into detail about how all the juices and sodas have sugar in them. Well, I was drinking orange juice every day, and I do not mean fresh squeezed orange juice. The orange juice was full of sugar, and it was concentrate.

First, I stopped drinking orange juice, and second, I stopped drinking coffee because I would put lots of sugar and cream in the coffee. Giving up coffee was very difficult because I love to drink coffee in the morning. I stopped drinking the coffee and orange juice and within 2 weeks I lost 4 pounds. This was the moment that made me eliminate sugar all together for about 2 months, and I started to do research in the library and book stores. Most people do not know I did research, but I needed to do this to help me understand. Some of the same comments my brother experienced from other people I also experienced. People were asking questions about how I lost weight. I was so excited; it made me want to lose more. People said, "You look really good and your face too." I knew it was the weight loss. The reason my face looked differently was because I lost weight in my face also.

Needless to say, I was able to lose 17 pounds. The good news is I have been able to keep it off. I eat cake, cookies, candy, and I drink juice/soda/coffee but in moderation. I drink mostly water with all my meals daily. This is how I have been able to not gain the weight back. I am so thankful.

I was Addicted to this Drug

VOLUME 2

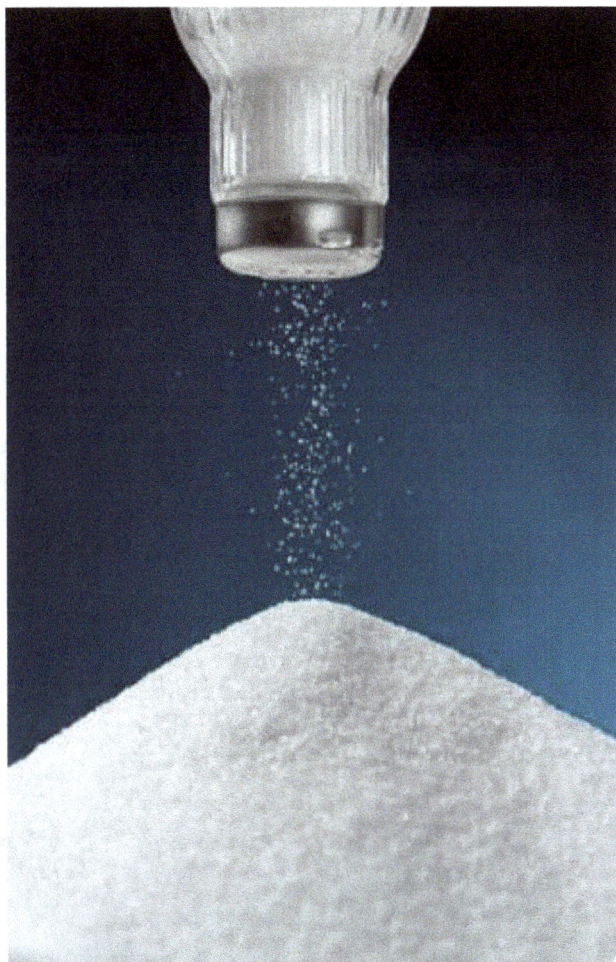

Chapter 1

Sugar's Deadly Twin

Earlier, I wrote about the deadly health consequences of eating refined sugar. It is without a doubt the number one enemy of things we consume. Sugar is produced by the tons, and we consume it by the tons. This process will not stop any time soon, so be aware. What I did not know was sugar has a twin killer I wasn't aware of. This product comes in the form of white crystals also. Most people have it in their kitchen cabinets. I'm sure you know the answer, right?

It is funny because I had no idea how much of salt freaks we are. I can understand us being addicted to sugar because everyone likes the taste of something sweet. But the surprising thing I found is that salt is basically in everything also, but it is disguised under different names. What is even worse is it only takes a small amount of salt to do much damage throughout the body.

Before we start, let's go back in time and see when in the U.S. the eating of salt became practical. Now of course we know no one invented this white crystal but nature itself. It is formed in the sea or in salt mines deep inside the earth. Since humanity has roamed this planet, they have been using salt for many purposes. In ancient times, they ate it also but in minimal amounts. One of its main purposes was to preserve food, such as meats. This method works better than our common refrigerator.

Salt was used for many spiritual purposes as well. It was used to bless weddings, and this ritual is done to this day. It was also used to preserve mummies in different parts of the world. Many religious cultures use salt in rituals to get rid of demons.

Cultivating these white crystals was in very high demand just a few hundred years ago. It was more valuable than it is today. Before the Americans were westernized, the Indians traded these valuable crystals on a routinely basis. These priceless crystals could be traded for anything.

Salt mining traditions continued as the pioneers expanded their way throughout the western frontier. The trading power of salt would decline, but it would always be a hot commodity. Humans will always have a connection for it is a great natural mineral of this planet. Over time, the usage of these crystals has grown to numerous heights. There are more than a few hundred different ways that people use it. Here is a short list that might be beneficial to your everyday life.

Salt's Purposes

1. Its most significant use is on our highways in the U.S. It is used as a de-icing compound for concrete surfaces.

2. For an emergency grease fire, pour salt over the fire. Never use water.

3. Rinse a scratchy eye with salt water

4. Salt and lemon juice removes mildew

5. Warm water and salt cleans drains

6. Use as a polish to cleanse brass and silver

7. Pour salt over spills inside the oven while it is still warm. Spills will go away easily.

8. Sprinkle salt on washed skillets. Warm it for a couple of minutes and wipe. Food will no longer stick to skillet.

9. Remove coffee stain from cups.

10. Pour into places to discourage ants from gathering there.

11. Clean the back of the iron with salt.

12. Wash greens and lettuce with salt water. This will keep them from withering.

13. Test eggs by placing them in salt water. Fresh eggs will float, and bad eggs will sink to the bottom.

Chapter 2

Table Salt

Since ancient times, we have been using this white substance in our diets. However, the quality of this mineral has diminished tremendously. Back in time, the tribes allowed the minerals to sun dry naturally just like they did all their foods. They weren't consuming a lot of salt in ancient times, but with the misinformation of knowledge in the last hundred years, we have consumed salt at alarming rates.

It has diminished down to what is known as table salt, which is composed of sodium chloride. All living creatures require the two components in minor quantities. The key word is minor, which means a very small amount. Health experts recommend that people should limit their intake of this mineral. Despite the recommendations, how did the American household end up with their cabinets full of sodium?

Most of the salt people have in their kitchen is table salt and iodized salt. Both of these happen to be heavily refined. In the early 19th century, additives, such as magnesium carbonate and potassium iodide, came into the equation. Table salt is more heavily processed to eliminate trace minerals and additives are added to prevent clumping. Iodized salt is basically table salt with iodine added to it. The added iodine is beneficial, but perhaps it is the only beneficial part of this harmful salt.

Since the U.S. became westernized, the salt intake grew unfortunately, and to this day, this white crystal remains in our cabinets waiting to harm us every time we sprinkle it on our foods. Just like the sugar sitting in our kitchen, salt is being used as a weapon against us.

Ever since we started consuming more of this product, our health has declined. And using the word declined is probably an understatement. Our health has been devastated, for we have suffered countless casualties, but the devastation continues and the casualties have rapidly increased since the early 19th century. This is when table salt was introduced as a condiment and for health reasons. Health advisors added iodine to salt and told us it was beneficial for our bodies. **Is this really the truth?**

This mineral would go on to become a drug to the American household. People couldn't consume cooked food unless it had a salty taste. The history of my family is of a black culture, so I am a witness to this kind of food. My culture consumes delicious dishes known as soul food. This is truly a great tasting food, but it is saturated with sodium. The fried chicken is full of salt, the macaroni and cheese is full of salt, and I'm not going to mention how much salt is in the baby back ribs. These are just a couple of soul food items. There are many more tasty items, and they are all contaminated. A couple of days eating such foods will turn the body into a walking salt mine.

If people think that this is just a problem for the black cultures, they are highly mistaken. In America, all the cultures have adapted to a disorder for sodium-based foods. We are addicted, and this addiction leads us to the hospital. Once we get there, we are subject to all kinds of treatments, and then we get multiple pills for our thrills.

So the question is why is all this so-called sodium in all our foods? The answer is because that some groups of people want it in all our foods. Some would call it a conspiracy. These people whoever they are want people to stay sick in my opinion. They must be powerful because they have convinced the food administration to allow harmful foods to be sold to the public. Or maybe this powerful group is none other than the food administration itself.

The main source of sodium in food these days comes in the form of monosodium glutamate (MSG). One of the reasons it is used is to enhance the taste of certain products. It has been known to effectively enhance the tastes of food no matter how cheap it is. This harmful product was created from seaweed in the early 1900's by a Japanese scientist. He isolated one element and extracted it from the seaweed plant, thus making it an unnatural salt. Salts are only natural in the form in which they were created. Thousands of years before this discovery, many different types of seaweed were used in their whole form in Japan, which was totally harmless.

Sodium is the reason our kids are obese. It wasn't until the 1940's that MSG would spread across the world at alarming rates. Along with it came many side effects at alarming rates! Since it can be produced so cheaply, most of the manufactures use it since the masses are unaware of the dangers that lurk within. These dangers are very much life threatening. I have listed a few of the symptoms below.

Joint pain

Irritable stomach

Flu

Migraines

Heart palpitations

Diarrhea

Panic attacks

Asthma

Depression

Anxiety

Rise or drop in blood pressure

Chapter 3

The Codes

I know many people, including myself, who said they were going to slow down on eating out at Asian eateries because of the high content of MSG. It's true they do use it a lot, but that is not the place one should be concerned about truthfully. Since the 70's, we have been poisoned with sodium with our American products. Most fast-food places carry high amounts of salty foods, and to my surprise maybe the biggest culprit is our grocery stores where MSG remains hidden under code names. Of course we are not told this, but it is coded with about 40 different names. This will probably increase because new chemicals are being introduced into food yearly.

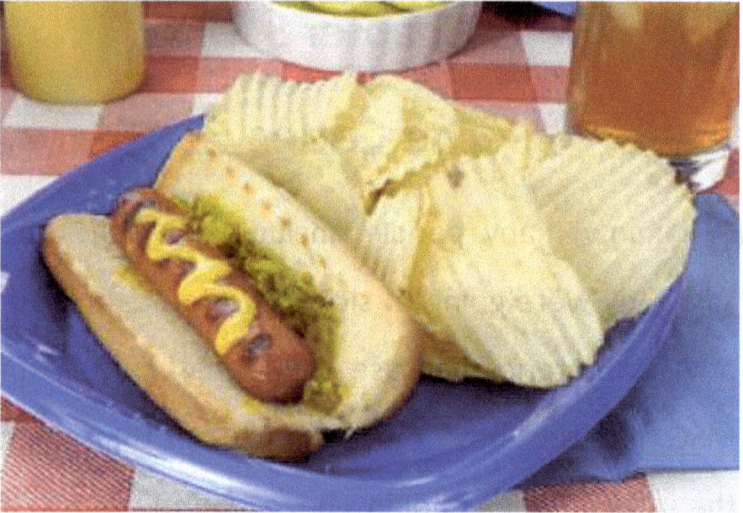

Coded MSG Ingredients

Yeast food

Glutamic Acid

Gelatin

Monopotassium glutamate

Soy protein

Calcium glutamate

Hydrolyzed (anything)

Magnesium glutamate

Soy protein isolate

Whey Protein Isolate

Whey protein

Accent

Calcium Caseinate

Natural Flavors

We have been hooked on this chemical monosodium glutamate for quite some time now. Manufactures have sneaked it into many of our common foods under different names. The reason is a manufacturer can put out a product and label it as having no MSG in which they have every right to do. Under a code name, they can package and sell it as being harmless. There is something wrong with this picture. It is a purely a clever scheme.

Coded Sodium Additives

Malt extract

Maltodextrin

Carrageenan

Barley malt

Xanthan

Gum

Flavoring (anything)

Soy sauce

Chicken stock

Broths

Pork flavoring

Bouillon

Pectin

Ultra pasteurized

Fermented

Processing Food is Salty. It is true, most packaged foods have high sodium contents. Like sugar, it is put in these foods for different reasons. First of all, it enhances the flavor of food like no other ingredient. Salt even brings out the taste in anything sweet. It helps prevent spoilage by slowing down the process of bacteria growth, yeast, and mold. Another reason it is used is to disguise all the chemical tastes in food that we cannot detect. It acts as a drug by dumbing down our taste buds.

The problem is not when one sprinkles salt on food he/she is preparing unless pouring large quantities. The problem is every time people open their cabinets, they start stuffing their faces with processed garbage, far too much to keep the body out of harm's way.

Since we are not taught, we don't have a clue how much sugar and sodium we consume daily.

I was Addicted to this Drug

Chapter 4

If You are Addicted to Salt, You are Addicted to Sugar

Many of our processed foods contain a high amount sodium and sugar combined. They come in the form of chemical salts and chemical sugars. In other words, they come under code names. This is the real reason why so many of us are addicted to what is called junk food. For example, have you ever noticed a kid with a big bag of potato chips? They can't seem to put it down until just about all the chips are crushed down into their bellies.

Sodium is the Reason Why Kids are Obese. I never really paid attention to this until examining my son and his taste for chips, especially the chips that is really spicy and flavorful. I would watch him and his friends devour big bags at a time.

Now keep in mind, this was before I studied anything about salt. My deep thoughts were telling me something is in chips that weren't there before. It's amazing how the instincts tell us things that can be so true. Soon after that, I noticed a boom of all the major companies producing some kind of spicy chip. I knew something was drawing the kids toward this processed food.

What I found was that they boosted up the sodium chemicals to enhance the taste buds once again. They're just doing what they always do: slip some more products in their foods. The amounts of sodium now being used are at alarming rates.

Doctors recommend that adults eat no more than 1 teaspoon a day of salt. Well, how are people supposed to achieve something that they are not prepared for? One can't prepare because they don't have a clue that they are consuming sodium all day long. Oh yes, let's look into foods that contain the drug salt. Then ask yourself if you are consuming more than 1 teaspoon of salt a day.

Processed foods that contain high amounts of sodium:

Chips

Tortillas

Ketchup

Mayonnaise

Miracle whip

Energy drinks

Bread

Energy bars

Cheese

Salad dressing

Pizza

Soy/teriyaki sauce

Fast food

Lasagna

Noodles

Cereal

Canned soups

Olives

Vegetable juice

Canned beans

Most sauces

Crackers

Processed meats

Smoked meat

Canned meat

Processed frozen foods

Pot pies

As you can see on the list, these are common foods that most of us eat daily. We tend to regularly eat pizza and processed chicken wings. The same day, we eat fries covered in ketchup. Let's not forget about the big bag of chips we eat from morning until nightfall. What about the sausage and eggs you had for breakfast?

Of course, many of us have high blood pressure. It's not by mistake but by design. The design is to keep us hooked on sodium-based foods. Maybe the conspiracy is to control the population of people by suppressing the conditions of people. This is exactly what salt does to us in many ways. The overeating of this chemical causes us to have many deficiencies in the body. Therefore, it is killing the cells in our body at a rapid pace.

At the end of the day, there is a control factor based upon money that is keeping such a hold on us. Whether the particular food is at the grocery store or the fast-food chain, the goal is to get people dependent on as many products as possible. They know scientifically, people can become addicted to chemical salts and sugars.

Continuously, products are advertised in papers to constantly remind us to buy them. On television, there are millions spent on the pushing of products with high amounts of sodium. They know our taste buds are so desensitized that we cannot tell when something is too salty. This is when the conspiracy starts. Sodium puts us in the place we call hospitals. The hospitals get money by pushing another product to us called medicine. The twist comes in the story when the doctor tells us to lower our salt intake. This is a good thing, and it sounds so easy. The problem is refined salt is in many of the products under coded names. The deception is when we get home we stop pouring salt on food at home, and we think we have the problem fixed. We don't understand the coded words of the refined salt. We don't understand what products contain salt.

Then of course, we wonder why we are not getting any better in health. How are we supposed to keep money in our pockets when we are constantly purchasing so many salty products?

We deteriorate in health; then, we go pay the doctors to fix us. So in the end, you end up paying out money in two different ways. The first way is the product; the second way is the doctor bill.

This information is not a scare tactic but an aware tactic. It is simply our reality. The choice is yours whether you want to continuously shove too much salt down your mouths. I just know it would be beneficial for you and your family if the sodium intakes are lowered, and by doing so, your medical problems will also be decreased.

We only have one body, so take heed of what you put into it. You are what you eat. The truth of the matter is we really only need the salt that is naturally in fruits and vegetables. The table salt in your cabinet is unnecessary. The table salt in your cabinet is messing up your health. There is no health more beneficial that what Mother Nature has provided us with.

I am not a doctor nor do I want to be. The best doctor in my opinion is knowledge. Take control of your life and make a change. Don't get me wrong. I thank God for hospitals and doctors. We do need them, but we could need them much less if we would educate ourselves.

Closing Remarks

I want everyone to know the most important thing about this book is that hopefully this will be new information to a few people out there. It would be amazing if the information in this book helped someone to deal with one of his/her medical conditions. I know I can help someone out there.

God bless everyone,

Robert

I believe this book is a wake-up call, and I encourage people to do their own research.

God bless everyone,

Demetrice